KRISHA MARIE

Happy Curls

A step by step guide to healthy happy curls

This book was professionally typeset on Reedsy.
Find out more at reedsy.com

Contents

1

Introduction

Hello Curl Friends,

My name is Krisha Marie, I am the CEO of Crown Healing and I'm a highly sought-after hair stylist who has been in the beauty industry for over 10 years. I have a passion for creating beautiful hair transformations and I dedicate myself to giving my clients the best experience possible. I have also studied under and worked with some of the best texture experts in the industry. With my knowledge and expertise, I am able to create any look with precision and accuracy. I am also a global educator, traveling the world to teach other hairstylists how to work with natural textures. I am super passionate about education and proud to be a facilitator for other artists in my industry. With my wealth of experience, I am always learning and striving to master my craft.

I have dedicated myself to helping the curl community to feel confident in embracing their natural hair . That is why I am sharing my knowledge with all of you. From start to finish, this guide will simplify your styling and give you the knowledge you need to embrace your natural hair and to give you the confidence in wearing your Crown. You will learn everything you need to know from washing, styling and even what products to use. It is my ultimate goal to help heal any trauma you might have from having textured hair and to help you to embrace your natural hair. This book is for men, women and parents of children with textured hair. I hope you enjoy it!

2

Embracing your natural hair

Congratulations!! You are now on your curly hair journey! Curly hair can be challenging at times, but with the right care and attention, it can also be absolutely stunning. So take a deep breath, trust the process, and enjoy every step of your curly hair journey. Most importantly, embrace your natural curls and celebrate their unique beauty. If you are just starting on your journey just know it takes time to get your hair back to health. It's not going to happen overnight, you are going to have some bad hair days, so give yourself some grace. If you are a parent learning your child's hair then great job for taking the initiative to teach your child to love their hair.

From my experience, many clients come to me for the first time after waiting 1-2 years to cut their hair, because let's face it , there are not a lot of people we trust with our hair. Trust me I get it. Your hair has been the same length for as long as you can remember so cutting it will only make it shorter. You are growing it out! So you don't want it cut, or you just cut it yourself because the last stylist who cut it , cut it way too short.

While yes , this is true, cutting will make it shorter but NOT cutting it will keep it at the length it is and it's probably looking dry and see through at the bottom. And because you haven't cut your hair in awhile it's going to continue to break off, look thin, flat and not grow. The only way to fix that is to find someone you trust (preferably a stylist that specializes in curls) and cut off the dead ends. Sometimes only a few inches is needed to help grow your hair but others might need a big chop to start fresh. Especially for those with heat damage or chemical damage or if you are growing out your relaxer. I Know it can seem scary that's why it is important to do your research on the best stylist for you. If a big chop is too scary then cut as much as you can to get it as healthy as you can faster. Now once you do your cut it's important to keep up with your trims about every 3-4 months. You have to trim a tree for the fruit to grow , same goes for your hair! I promise that your hair will grow faster and fuller just by keeping up with your trims. They call it a journey for a reason. But if you stick to it, your curls will grow happy and healthy.

All curls are not created equal. What works for one person might not work for the next, so it's important to understand your curl type. Also it is very common for you to have more than one curl type on your head. So what is a curl type? There are a few charts and texture keys that can help you with typing out your curls, but the purpose of this book is to simplify it so you understand . So I put it into 3 categories. Waves, curls and coils.

Wavy hair is a type of hair that is characterized by its natural loose or defined S waves. This type of hair is neither completely straight nor curly, but falls somewhere in between. The wavy texture can range from subtle and soft to more defined and prominent, depending on the person's genetics and hair care routine. Waves grow down from the head which means less frizz since your natural oils can freely travel through the hair. Most wavy hair clients complain of lack of volume.

Curly hair is a type that's characterized by its spiral curl. This type of hair can be a loser big curl or a tighter smaller curl. Again depending on the person's genetics and hair care routine will determine softness or definition. There are two types of curls , ones that grow down from the head and creates a triangle shape or curls that grow horizontally witch creates a crescent shape , or ear muffs .Both have moderate to high volume in the hair but this also means that this curl type is prone to more frizz since the natural oil can't travel as freely as straight or wavy hair it can seem more dry. Most clients with curly hair complain of flatness at the crown and frizz.

Coily hair, on the other hand, is a hair type characterized by its tightly coiled or zigzag-shaped hair strands.Coily hair typically has a tighter curl pattern than curly hair,and its coils can range from small and tight to larger and looser . Coiled hair grows vertical from the head leaving the hair more prone to dryness and requires proper hydration and moisturization to prevent breakage and promote healthy hair growth. Coily hair can be more challenging to manage and style, as it can be prone to tangling and requires more effort to detangle and style. However this texture type has high volume and holds its shape. Most clients with this texture complain about shrinkage, definition and dryness. See chart below.

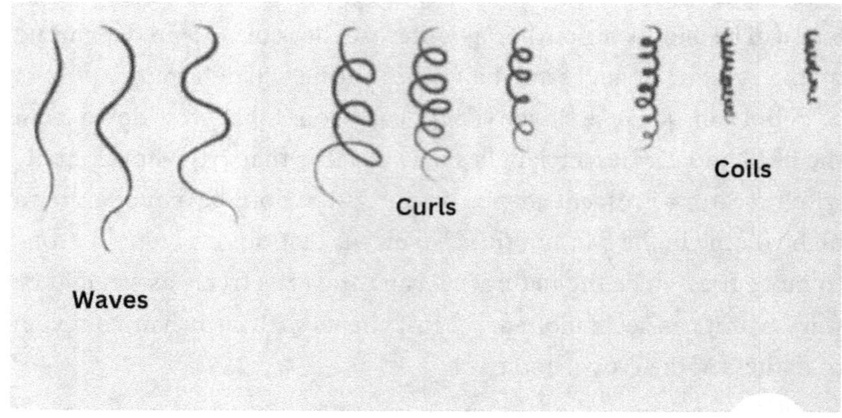

Now let's talk about the scalp. Scalp care is very important for maintaining healthy hair growth and preventing scalp infections or irritations. A buildup of dirt, oil and product residue on the scalp can clog hair follicles and hinder your hair growth and can also lead to dandruff or other scalp conditions. I always tell my clients healthy scalp means healthy hair. Our scalp is an extension of our skin so make sure you are exfoliating and massaging your scalp so you can stimulate the blood flow and promote healthy happy hair.

So Many of my clients come in and complain about hair loss but 9 times out of 10 is just natural shedding. Natural hair shedding is a normal and natural process that occurs as part of the hair growth cycle. It is estimated that on average, people shed between 50-100 hairs per day. With texture hair the hair strands don't fall off the head like straight hair. It tends to stay in the hair until it's washed. If you don't wash your hair everyday more times than not you will have days of natural shedding in your hair. Which can look scary in the shower, but most of the time there is no need to worry. However while some hair shedding is normal , excessive shedding may be a sign of an underlying health condition, such as thyroid issues or nutrient deficiencies. It's important to pay attention to your hair shedding patterns and consult with a healthcare provider if you notice sudden or excessive hair loss.

3

Cleansing your curls

Let's get into the wash day. Whether you got this book to learn your own hair or someone else, it's key to know that keeping your curls clean is crucial for maintaining healthy hair and a long-lasting hairstyle, especially for textured hair types. Now cleansing the curls doesn't mean you cleanse every time you style your curls, but definitely incorporate it in your routine. As you have heard me say before, texture hair is more prone to dryness and breakage due to its natural structure and how our natural oil can not travel through the hair. Product buildup, dirt and oil can clog the hair follicles, leading to scalp irritation and inhibiting healthy hair growth. Regularly washing your curls with a sulfate-free shampoo and conditioner not only removes buildup but also provides necessary moisture and hydration to the hair strands. This helps to prevent breakage and split ends , and allows for a defined and bouncy curl pattern. Additionally, a clean and healthy scalp promotes hair growth, which is essential for maintaining voluminous and healthy happy curls. By keeping your curls clean, you can ensure healthy , vibrant, and long lasting hair that looks and feels its best.

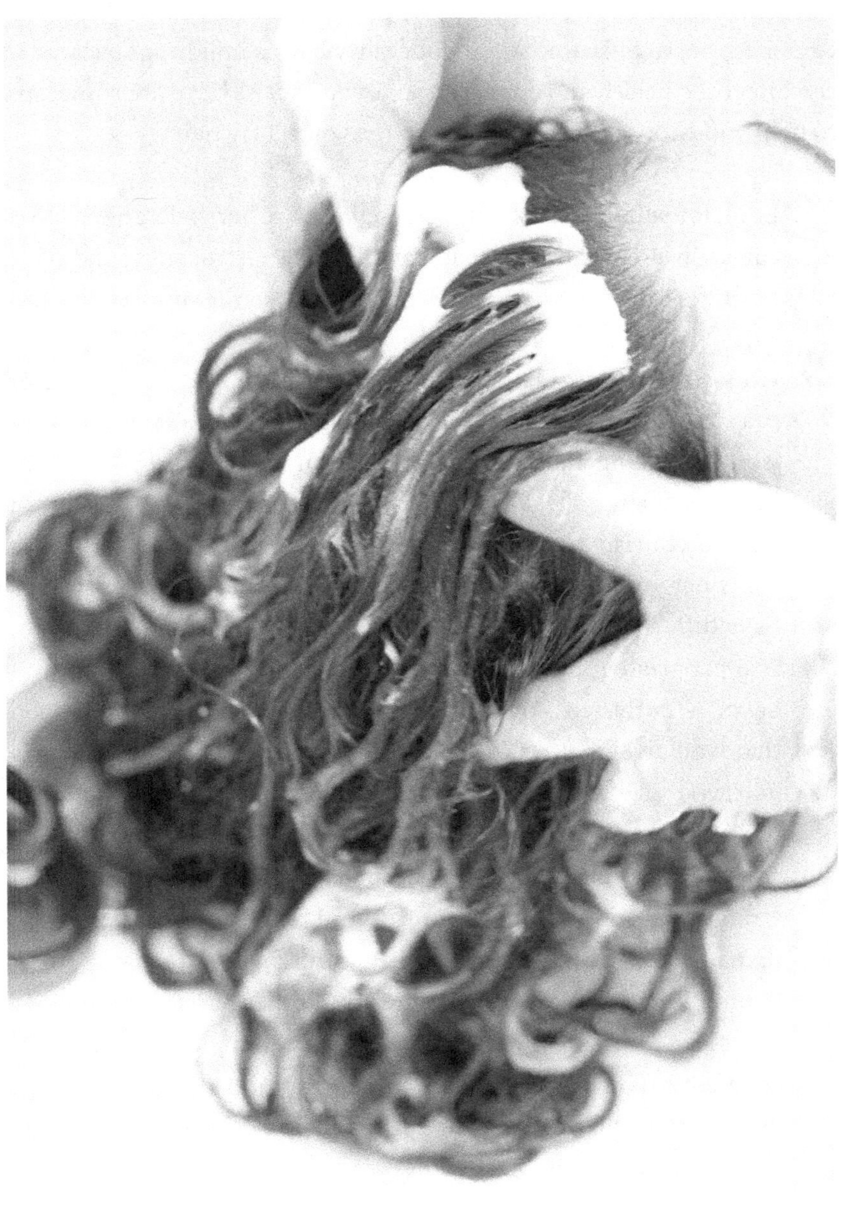

Choosing the right shampoo for your curly hair is important because it can affect the health and appearance of your curls. Here are some tips to help you choose the best shampoo for your curly hair:

1. Look for sulfate-free shampoos: Sulfates are harsh detergents that can strip curly hair of its natural oils and cause dryness and frizz. Look for shampoos that are labeled sulfate-free or contain mild surfactants that are gentle on the hair.

2. Choose moisturizing shampoos: Curly hair tends to be drier than straight hair, so it's important to choose a shampoo that is moisturizing and hydrating. Look for shampoos that contain ingredients like shea butter, coconut oil, or argan oil, which can help to nourish and moisturize your curls.

3. Consider your hair type and texture: Different types of curly hair have different needs, so it's important to choose a shampoo that is appropriate for your hair type and texture. For example, if you have fine curly hair, you may want to choose a lightweight shampoo that won't weigh your curls down. If you have thick, coarse curly hair, you may want to choose a shampoo that is richer and more hydrating.

4. Avoid harsh chemicals: Curly hair is often more delicate than straight hair, so it's important to avoid harsh chemicals that can damage or dry out your curls. Look for shampoos that are free from sulfates, parabens, phthalates, and other harsh chemicals.

5. Consider your lifestyle: If you live in a dry climate or swim frequently, you may want to choose a shampoo that is specifically designed to help protect your curls from the effects of chlorine or environmental stressors.

By considering these factors and experimenting with different shampoos, you can find the best shampoo for your curly hair that will help to keep your curls healthy, hydrated, and looking their best

Pre cleansing and do you need to do it? It depends on your hair and how often you wash it. A Pre cleanser is just that , a pre cleanse. It is a type of cleansing product that is used before shampooing your hair . It is designed to loosen up buildup and excess oil from your scalp and hair strands, allowing your shampoo to work more effectively. Pre- cleaners are applied to dry hair before getting in the shower. The product is massaged into the scalp and hair. I recommend pre cleansers to those of you who use a lot of products, have naturally oily hair or live a very active lifestyle. Also great for parents to do on their children before they shower. A pre cleanser will ensure a great start to effectively cleanse and nourish your hair, leaving it feeling clean, refreshed and healthy.

I am pretty sure you have been hearing about clarifying shampoo. It seems like it's the new big thing, but it's been around for a long time. Why is it so important? It's important to clarify your hair because curly hair tends to be more prone to buildup of product residue, dirt and oil that can weigh down the curls and make them lose their natural bounce and volume. Clarifying helps to remove this buildup, leaving the hair feeling clean and refreshed.Clarifying also helps to prevent dandruff and scalp irritation, which can be more common in curly hair due to its texture.

As for how often you should clarify, it depends on your hair type and how much product you use. If you use a lot of heavy styling products,it may be necessary to clarify once a week or every two weeks. However if you have drier hair that isn't prone to build up, you may only need to clarify once a month. It's important to pay attention to how your hair looks and feels and adjust your clarifying routine accordingly. Over-clarifying can strip the hair of its natural oils and cause dryness, so it's best to find a balance that works for your individual hair type. If you're still not sure, ask your hairstylist..

Another product you may have heard of is a cleansing conditioner or co- wash. I only recommend using a co wash if you are someone that washes your hair more frequently. A cleansing conditioner is a hair care product that combines the cleansing properties of a shampoo with the conditioning benefits of a conditioner. It is designed to gently cleanse the hair without stripping it of its natural oils or causing dryness. Unlike traditional shampoos that contain harsh detergents that create a lot of foam and suds, cleansing conditioners do not lather as much or at all. The lack of foam might need some getting used to, but it does not mean that the product is less effective at cleaning the hair.

Finally, how to wash your hair. Yes there is a way to wash textured hair. Textured hair is fragile hair because of all the dips and curves of the hair structure but it's even more fragile when it's wet. That's why I prefer my clients to dry their hair vs air dry. But we will get to that later on in the book. I like to teach my clients to use their hands when they detangle. I feel as if it gives you more control vs a comb or brush which can tear the hair. For those of you with coiled hair using a brush before the shower can help detangle and make shampooing easier. You want to brush from the ends and work your way up. Also it takes longer, meaning you're actually washing your hair and not rubbing it in real fast then washing it out. You want to take your hand and comb thru or rake in a downward motion to wash, detangle and smooth the hair. If You put your hair on the top of your head and move it all around like the herbal essence commercial then you're only causing tangles and frizz. I tell my clients that the styling begins in the shower. Start smoothing down that cuticle and detangle so that styling will be much easier (like the picture below).

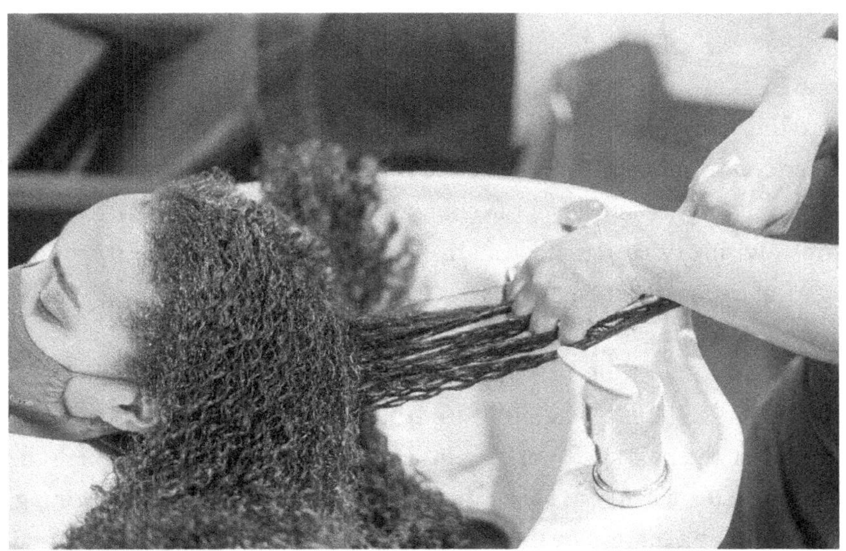

Next you are going to want to condition in the same manner as the shampoo, in a downward motion raking through to detangle. Conditioning and deep conditioning are two important steps in your hair care routine that can help to improve the overall health and appearance of the hair, while both are beneficial, they serve different purposes. Conditioner is a product that is used after shampooing to help detangle, moisturize and smooth the hair. Because you have already started detangling with the shampoo it is going to be a lot easier when you start to style. I recommend using a conditioner every time you wash your hair. It's meant to seal the cuticle of the hair which can prevent damage and breakage.

Deep conditioning on the other hand is a more intense form of conditioning that is designed to provide extra nourishment and repair to the hair. Deep conditioners contain higher concentrations of ingredients such as proteins, vitamins, and oils that penetrate deeper into the hair shaft to repair and strengthen the hair from the inside out . Deep conditioning can be done once a week or once a month, depending on the hair type and level of damage. It is particularly beneficial for those with dry or damaged hair, as it can help to restore the hair's natural moisture and elasticity.

Steam is another tool that can be used along with the deep conditioner. Steam is a small molecule of water that is small enough to be able to penetrate the hair shaft pushing in water conditioner or treatment on the hair. Steam can provide a range of benefits , including moisturizing, softening, and increasing the elasticity of the hair. When hair is exposed to steam, the heat and moisture can help to open up the hair cuticle, allowing for better absorption of moisture and nutrients.

4

Conditioning your curls

Next you are going to want to condition in the same manner as the shampoo, in a downward motion raking through to detangle. Conditioning and deep conditioning are two important steps in your hair care routine that can help to improve the overall health and appearance of the hair, while both are beneficial, they serve different purposes. Conditioner is a product that is used after shampooing to help detangle, moisturize and smooth the hair. Because you have already started detangling with the shampoo it is going to be a lot easier when you start to style. I recommend using a conditioner every time you wash your hair. It's meant to seal the cuticle of the hair which can prevent damage and breakage.

Deep conditioning on the other hand is a more intense form of conditioning that is designed to provide extra nourishment and repair to the hair. Deep conditioners contain higher concentrations of ingredients such as proteins, vitamins, and oils that penetrate deeper into the hair shaft to repair and strengthen the hair from the inside out . Deep conditioning can be done once a week or once a month, de;pending on the hair type and level of damage. It is particularly beneficial for those with dry or damaged hair, as it can help to restore the hair's natural moisture and elasticity.

Steam is another tool that can be used along with the deep conditioner. Steam is a small molecule of water that is small enough to be able to penetrate the hair shaft pushing in water conditioner or treatment on the hair. Steam can provide a range of benefits , including moisturizing, softening, and increasing the elasticity of the hair. When hair is exposed to steam, the heat and moisture can help to open up the hair cuticle, allowing for better absorption of moisture and nutrients.

5

Styling your curls

Let's talk about products. Products are our friends. Using the right products can help keep moisture in the hair and help give you a long lasting style. Knowing if your hair is fine or course will give you an idea which products to use. Most curly hair clients have fine hair but high density meaning they have a lot of hair and mistakenly think they have coarse hair ultimately using the wrong products. You want to stay clear of oils or heavy butters, because they do not moisturize the hair. As far as what products to use you want to use products that are best for your type of texture , things to consider are hydration, weight and hold. For example if you have wavy hair most likely you are going to need a mouse or gel to help with hold , curl cream can be too heavy and weigh down the hair. For curlier hair I love using a cream or mousse for moisture and then a little gel for some hold. With coily hair a cream leave in is recommended and then a foam or gel for hold.But again, what works for one might not work for another so playing around with different products and distribution is best.

Step 1 to styling . You want to start off with your hair really wet. You don't want it to be sopping wet because that will dilute the products but you do want your hair wet enough to where you hear a squishy sound when you scrunch. It's best to style your hair right out of the shower. I always keep a water bottle handy in case the hair starts to dry. I tell my clients if your hair looks frizzy when it's wet then it's going to look frizzy when it's dry. Water is key to juicy looking curls.

Step 2, apply your leave-in conditioner first, a light spray leave-in is recommended for fine hair and a cream is recommended for thicker hair. Next Section your hair in 1 inch sections . I tell my clients if they take their time styling their hair on day one then they will most likely have a style that lasts them longer than if they were to rush this process. Next apply something for hold , for finer hair I like using gel or mouse, or curl creams and gels for thicker hair. When applying Products it is recommended to always apply mid-shaft to the ends. This technique is so you don't apply too much product on the roots. This is where I teach my client to use a brush. A denim brush is perfect to brush the product through the hair Tthis will ensure proper distribution of the product and also helps to clump your curls. If you don't have a brush you can use the rake and shake method, Where you use your hands like a rake to clump the hair and then give it a good shake to encourage the curl. After the products are distributed through the hair and the hair is clumped you want to make sure that you don't touch your hair at all until it's about 80% dry.

Protip; Brush under vs over to create more volume at the root.

If you have bangs, you are going to want to section them out forward before drying.

Before drying, I like to have my client flip upside down and then I'll scrunch in some foam or mouse. If it seems as though the hair is super saturated with products and water , take a microfiber towel and scrunch the hair to encourage the curl and to take out some excess moisture before we dry.

Now it's time to dry. Diffusing and air drying are two popular ways to dry curly hair. Diffusing is a technique where you use a diffuser attachment on your hair dryer to gently dry your curls. The diffuser helps to distribute the heat evenly and reduce frizz, while also enhancing your natural curl pattern. Air drying is simply allowing your hair to dry naturally without the use of any heat or tools. This is a low-maintenance option that can be a good choice for those who prefer a more natural look.

So which is better? The answer depends on your personal preference, hair type, and lifestyle. If you have the time and prefer a more natural look, air drying may be a good option. If you need to dry your hair quickly or want to enhance your natural curl pattern, diffusing may be a better choice. Ultimately, both methods can be effective if done properly, and you can experiment to find the best option for your hair

I recommend my clients to dry their hair as much as possible using a heat protectant. As you heard me say before, your hair is more fragile when it's wet so drying will ensure that you have less breakage and frizz. You are going to want to start off with a hover like the photo below. Do not start on your ends. Your ends are pores and typically dry the fastest so always hover and start at the root then work your way to the ends. If you want encouragement of the curls then you will want to place your ends in the diffuser and scrunch up to help your curls create volume . If you already have tons of volume and don't want shrinkage then you can continue to hover or sit under a hooded dryer.

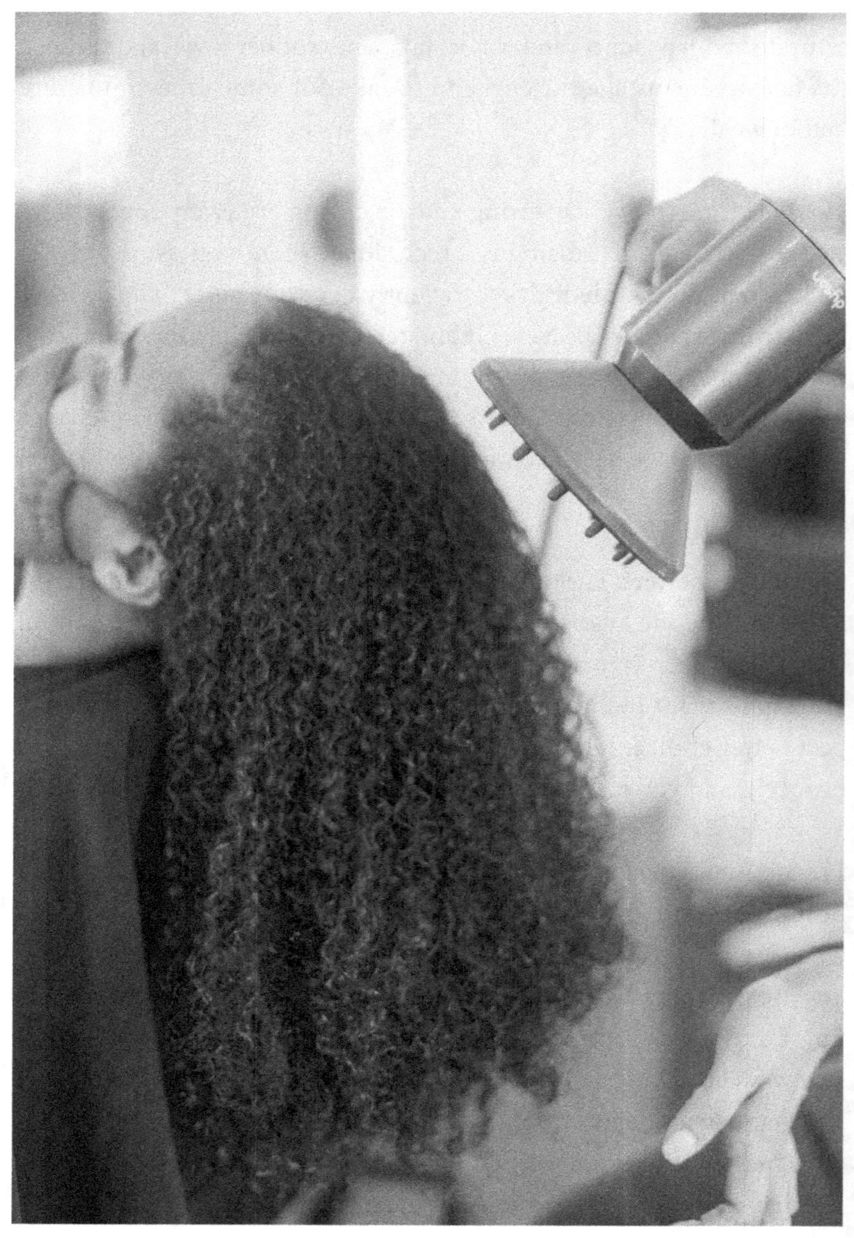

When diffusing, keep the settings of the dryer on low heat and low pressure of the air. This will help ensure that your hair won't frizz. Starting off too hot will take moisture out of the hair before the products can do their job. After a good 5 minutes you can turn up the heat but always keep the pressure on low, again making sure you don't touch the hair. When diffusing it's best to dry the hair to about 80- 90 % dry. Once it's 80-90% dry that's when you can go in and start separating the clumped hair. This will give volume to the hair. Make sure to use a serum or oil on your hands while separating the curls to ensure that you don't frizz the hair. Once you separate, continue to dry til it's 100% dry before fluffing or breaking the cast.

What does it mean to break the cast? A cast is when your hair is 100% dry and feels hard and crunchy from the product. That is called a cast and it ensures a long lasting style. However we want to break the cast so your hair feels soft and not hard. There are a few ways to go about breaking the cast . You can flip upside down and give your hair a good shake being cautious of not raking through your curls. Another option is using the dryer at the root to loosen up the curls.You can also leave the cast and let it naturally break from everyday life or when you sleep. This is best for individuals who want their style to last all week. Which brings me to sleeping and how you should sleep with your hair.

Honestly I don't do anything with my hair when I sleep, I always felt as though a good night's rest was more important than keeping my hair nice. But if you are wanting ways to protect your hair you can always wear it in a pineapple where you loosley wear your hair on top of your head using a silk scrunchy. You can also use a silk bonnet or silk pillowcase to help protect your hair from frizz.

Refreshing curly hair in the morning can be a quick and easy way to revive your curls and extend the life of your hairstyle. Here are some steps to refresh your curls:

1. Start by dampening your hair with water or a spray bottle filled with a water-based leave-in conditioner. This will help to rehydrate your curls and reactivate any styling products you applied the day before.

2. Apply a small amount of a lightweight styling product such as a curl refreshing spray or mousse to help define your curls and reduce frizz. Be sure to avoid heavy products that can weigh down your curls or make them feel greasy.

3. Use your fingers to scrunch your hair upwards, encouraging your curls to reform and bounce back into shape.

4. If your curls are still looking a bit flat, use a diffuser attachment on your hairdryer to gently dry your hair while scrunching it upwards. This will help to enhance your curls and create more volume.

5. Finish by using a small amount of oil or serum to smooth down any frizz or flyaways and add shine to your hair. You can also use a hairspray or a curl-defining gel to help set your curls and keep them in place throughout the day.

Remember that refreshing your curly hair in the morning is all about finding what works best for your hair type and texture. Don't be afraid to experiment with different products and techniques to find the perfect routine for your curls.

You are all done! Now it's time to get a routine going and to schedule your next haircut. Getting regular haircuts is essential for maintaining healthy, strong, and beautiful hair. Here is a reminder why:

1. Promoting hair growth: Cutting your hair regularly can actually promote hair growth. By removing the damaged ends of your hair, you are encouraging the hair to grow stronger and healthier. In addition, regular haircuts can also help to stimulate blood flow to the scalp, which can promote hair growth.

2. Maintaining style and shape: If you have a specific hairstyle, regular haircuts are essential for maintaining the style and shape. Over time, hair can become overgrown and lose its shape, making it harder to style. Regular haircuts can help to keep your hair looking its best and ensure that your hairstyle stays in place.

3. Managing hair texture: Hair texture can change over time, becoming coarser, finer, or more unruly. Regular haircuts can help to manage these changes by removing the damaged or uneven parts of the hair, leaving you with a smoother, more manageable texture.

4. Boosting confidence: A fresh haircut can make you feel more confident and put-together. Regular haircuts can help to maintain your hair's health and appearance, leaving you feeling more confident and ready to take on the day.

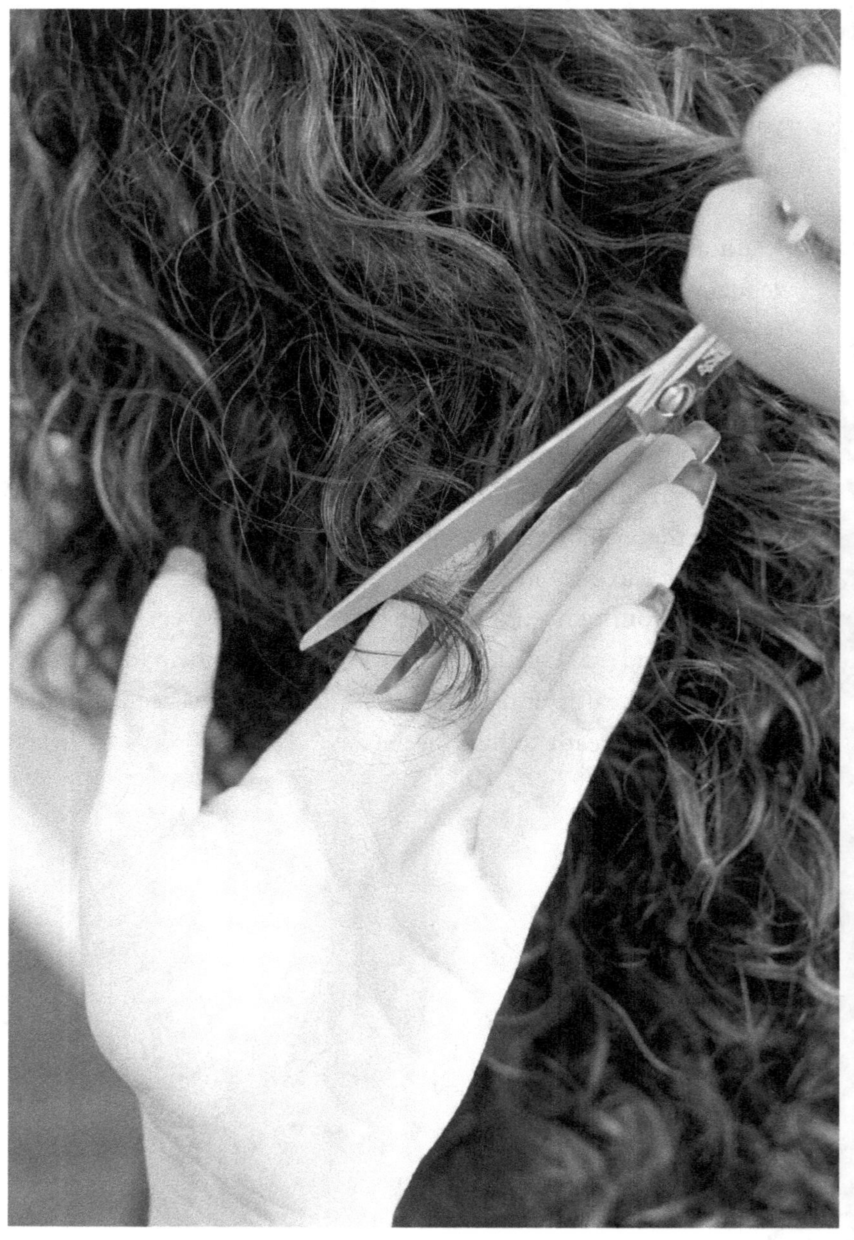

25

6

Conclusion

In summary, getting regular haircuts is important for maintaining the health and appearance of your hair. By preventing split ends, promoting hair growth, maintaining style and shape, managing hair texture, and boosting confidence, regular haircuts are an essential part of any hair care routine.

Understanding curly hair and how to properly care for it can make all the difference in achieving healthy, beautiful, and manageable curls. Throughout this book, we have explored the unique challenges and characteristics of curly hair, and dived into the various techniques and products that can help to enhance its natural beauty.

From embracing your natural texture and using the right shampoo and conditioner, to incorporating deep conditioning treatments and protective styling, there are a multitude of strategies that can help to maintain and nourish curly hair. It's important to remember that no two curls are alike, and finding the right routine for your individual hair type and texture may require some trial and error. Ultimately, the key to healthy and vibrant curls is embracing and loving your natural hair, and taking the time to care for it properly. With patience, consistency and a willingness to experiment, anyone can achieve gorgeous, bouncy curls that are the envy of all.

I want to thank all my beautiful loyal clients who trust me with their Crown and to all my mentors over the years who have taught and inspired me.

I am constantly learning and will always have the passion to teach others what I know.

Thank you! Love & Light,
  Krisha Marie
  www.krishamarie.com
  @krishastylesyou

P.s I would genuinely be grateful if you can take the time to leave a quick review on amazon.

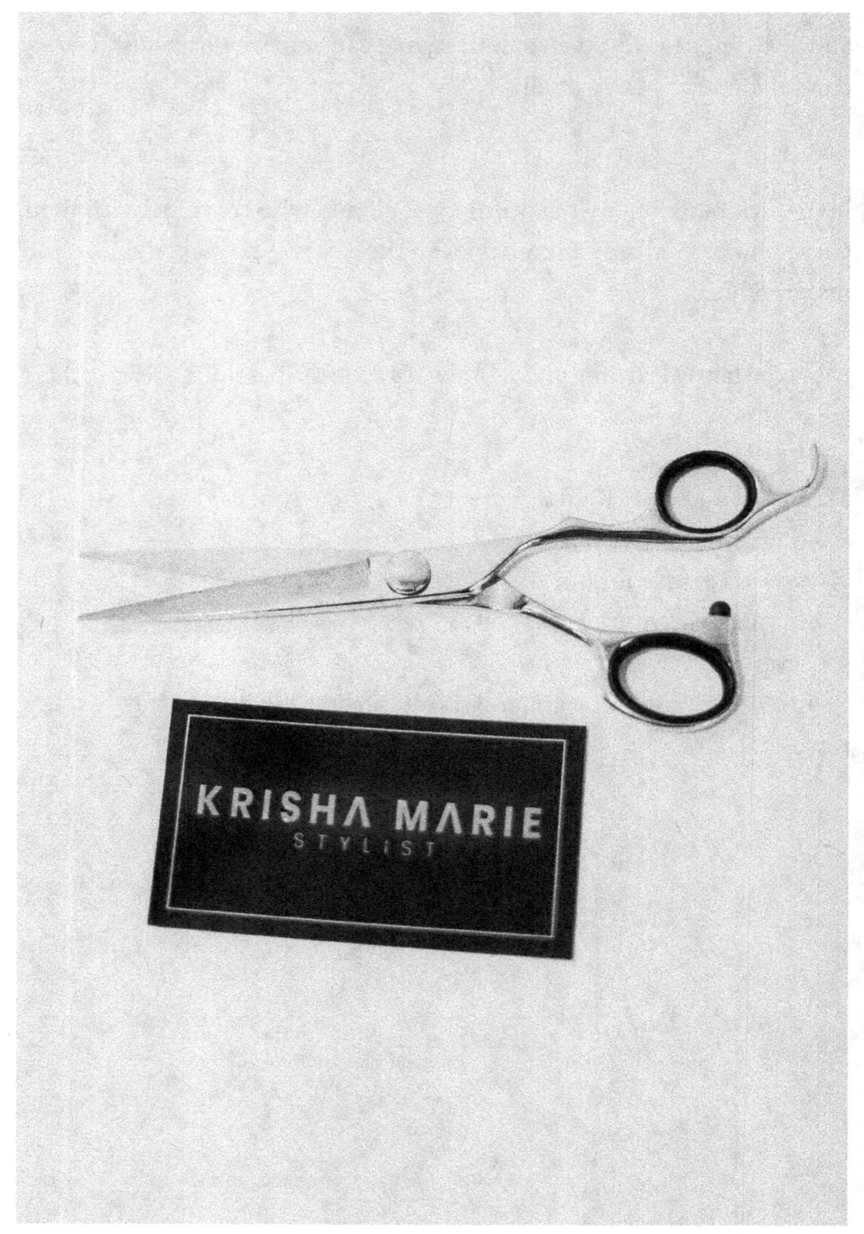
KRISHA MARIE
STYLIST

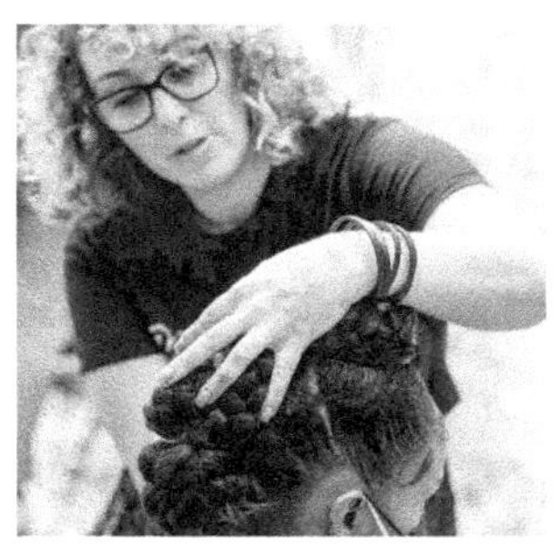

About the Author

Krisha is a highly sought-after hair stylist who has been in the beauty industry for over 10 years. She has a passion for creating beautiful hair transformations and is dedicated to giving her clients the best experience possible. With her knowledge and expertise, she is able to create any look with precision and accuracy. She is also a global educator, traveling the world to teach other hairstylists how to work with natural textures. Krisha is passionate about education and is proud to be a facilitator for other artists in her industry. With her wealth of experience, she is always learning and striving to master her craft.

Krisha is dedicated to providing a unique and luxurious experience for all of her clients. She is passionate about helping her clients feel confident in embracing their natural hair texture, and uses her expertise to create looks that will make them feel their best. From start to finish, she provides a personalized service that will help you heal any trauma behind textured hair, and show the world your natural crown.

You can connect with me on:

🌐 https://www.krishamarie.com